Brain Tumor Surgery and Anesthesia

Hala Goma, professor of Anesthesia, Cairo University

Table of contents

1. Introduction

Anesthesia has a great responsibility in brain tumor surgery; it may be in some times the longest role in brain tumor team. Preparative role in form of preparation of the patient, intraoperative management, post-operative care. The great price and challenge when the

Patient is systemically and neuro surgically stable, and leaving the hospital happy.

2. Mortality risk for elective brain tumor surgery

2.1 Impairment of general health by disease, or requiring surgery.

2.2 Ischemic heart disease.

2.3 Chronic lower Respiratory tract Infection.

2.4 Cardiac failure.

2.5 Obesity Impaired renal function.

2.6 Diabetes.

3. Preoperative evaluation

3.1 Aim of preoperative evaluation

To obtain pertinent information about the patient's medical history and physical and mental

Conditions, in order to determine which tests and consultations are needed.

Guided by patient choices and the risk factors uncovered by the medical history, to choose the care plans to be followed.

To obtain informed consent.

To educate the patient about anesthesia, perioperative care, and pain treatments in the hope of reducing anxiety and facilitating recovery.

To make perioperative care more efficient and less expensive.

To utilize the operative experience to motivate the patient to more optimal health and thereby improve perioperative and/or long-term outcome.

3.2 Table 1. Medical problems discovered on pre anesthetic evaluation that could prompt a change in patient management History Point Concern/Area to Evaluate Anesthesia Plans That May Require

Extra Time

Airway perceived   intubate. Airway; prior anesthesia, outcomes. Help.

Asthma Pulmonary disease Optimize therapy; use bronchodilators; possibly extubation during deep anesthesia.

Diabetes, insulin dependent.

Endocrine, metabolic, diabetes

Discuss insulin management with patient and primary care doctor; monitor blood glucose intra operatively; determine presence of autonomic neuropathy and plan management appropriately, such as administration of metoclopramide and PACU or ICU stay.

Drug abuse Social history Consider HIV testing; prescribe medications to avoid withdrawal symptoms in perioperative period.

Gastro esophageal gastrointestinal disease: hiatus

Administer H2 antagonists or oral antacids and **reflux or hiatus hernia.** Hernia. Use rapid-sequence induction of anesthesia; or use awake intubation techniques and obtain appropriate equipment.

Heart disease:

Risk of subacute bacterial Endocarditis

Antibiotic prophylaxis.

Arrange for antibiotic administration 1h prior

Valve disease, to surgery.

Malignant hyperthermia

Prior anesthetic/surgical history Obtain clean anesthesia machine; use

History, family history, or suspected potential history

Appropriate technique and precautions; have agents to treat Malignant hyperthermia available.

Monoamine oxidase inhibitors.

CNS: psychiatric/medication Discontinue therapy preoperatively if patient is not suicidal; plan for perioperative pain therapy.

Pacemaker or Cardiovascular disease: Evaluate cause of pacemaker

Implementation;

Automatic Electrocardiogram. Obtain repolarizing equipment or Magnet; use **implantable cardiac defibrillator.** Electro cautery with altered position; use bipolar electro cautery.

Neuropathy.

Peripheral motor CNS disease: neurologic deficit Avoid depolarizing muscle relaxants.

Pregnancy

Monitor fetal heart rate; use oral antacids; **uncertain** adjust induction of anesthesia; determine status

Pregnancy status of pregnancy.

Pulmonary disease: Use disposable breathing circuit or clean one.

Tuberculosis. Tuberculosis. Equipment; ensure adequate treatment of pulmonary TB.

3.3 Physical examination

Determination of arterial blood pressure in both arms, and in at least one arm 2 minutes after the patient assumes the upright position after lying down. (Third and fourth heart sounds).

Examination of the carotid and jugular pulses.

Examination of the chest and auscultation of the bases of the heart for subtle rales suggestive of congestive heart failure, or for rhonchi, wheezes, and other sounds indicative of lung disease. (Although history-taking may detect these symptoms that point to lung disease as accurately as auscultation.

Observation of the patient's walk for signs of neurologic disease and to assess back mobility and general health.

Examination of the eyes for abnormal movement and, along with the skin, for signs of jaundice, cyanosis, nutritional abnormalities, and dehydration.

The fingers are checked for clubbing.

Examination of the airway and mouth for neck mobility, tongue size, oral lesions, and ease of intubation.

Examination of the legs for bruising, edema, clubbing, mobility, sensation.

3.4 Preoperative surgical evaluation

The level of consciousness, neurological deficits and occurrence of seizures need to be noted.

The existence of intracranial space occupation and raised ICP (persistent headache, vomiting, and papilledema) must be evaluated.

Posterior fossa tumors may cause bulbar palsy and the lower cranial nerves should be examined for impairment of swallowing or laryngeal palsy. A history of repeated aspiration of stomach contents, perhaps with nocturnal bronchospasm, reveals laryngeal incompetence.

The assessment of supratentorial lesions is made considerably easier by the improvement in

Imaging techniques, CT scanning and MRI. These allow early, precise location of lesions and give some idea of the probable histological diagnosis. The scans should be examined to give information on:

☐ Size of mass;

☐ Ventricular distortion or CSF obstruction;

☐ Midline shift;

☐ Amount of edema;

☐ Degree of contrast enhancement;

☐ Proximity to venous sinus.

☐ the size of the mass depends partly on whether the tumor is developing in a silent or an eloquent area of the brain. Tumors in a silent area may grow so large before they present that they cause a very considerable compromise of intracranial dynamics.

☐ Assessment of the degree of intracranial space occupation is important; if there is more than 10 mm shift of the midline structures, for example, volatile agents should be used with care. The amount of edema may turn a relatively small lesion into a more serious problem.

☐ the degree of enhancement with intravenous radiographic contrast shows the degree of abnormal or damaged. Blood–brain barrier (BBB) in the lesion and it is through this damaged BBB that the contrast penetrated to the stroma of the tumor.

☐ a vascular tumor may have a low vascular resistance and frequently in angiography cerebral veins draining the tumor fill early, during the arterial or capillary phases of the angiogram, reflecting the fast flow. Such a tumor, especially if it is near one of the Venous sinuses, has the potential for causing major blood loss as resection is undertaken.

☐ the increasing availability of metabolic imaging such as PET, MR spectroscopy and single photon emission tomography (using thallium-201 which is specifically taken up by tumor cells but not by necrotic areas) will offer more precise information on the size and location of the tumor. Patients suspected of having an astrocytoma shouldundergo stereotactic biopsy prior to craniotomy to confirm the histological diagnosis.

3.5 Preoperative investigation

☐ Electrocardiogram (ECG).

ECG Abnormality.

T wave, ST segment, Arrhythmias, SVT or PVC, PAC, QRS, Q wave.

Ventricular conduction defects AV block, AV, atrioventricular; ECG, electrocardiogram;

LVH, Left ventricular hypertrophy; PAC, premature atrial contractions; PVC, premature ventricular contractions; SVT, supraventricular tachycardia.

☐ Chest Radiographs.

Tracheal deviation or compression; mediastinal masses; pulmonary nodules; a solitary lung mass; aortic aneurysm; pulmonary edema; pneumonia; atelectasis; new fractures of the vertebrae, ribs, and clavicles; dextrocardia; and cardiomegaly. However, a chest radiograph probably would not detect the degree of chronic lung disease requiring a change in anesthetic technique any better than would the history or physical examination.

□ **Echocardiography is indicated in ischemic, valvular, and pronged hypertension and diabetes.**

□ *Laboratory investigation:*

Hemoglobin, Hematocrit, and White Blood Cell Counts.

Blood Chemistries, Urinalysis, and Clotting Studies, fasting blood glucose, renal, hepatic functions, BUN, hepatitis markers for A and C for medico legal risk posed by post anesthetic ,jaundice .

□ **Preparation of blood transfusion:**

A large meningioma can be associated with heavy blood loss but for most craniotomies 2–4 units of blood are sufficient.

3.6 Preoperative investigation

Normal medication, especially anticonvulsants and antihypertensive drugs, should be continued until just before surgery. Sedative premedication may be desirable in order to allay anxiety. Respiratory depression with subsequent hypercarbia should be avoided, especially in the presence of raised ICP. For this reason we avoid opiates and usually prescribe 10–20 mg of temazepam or 10–15 mg, diazepam, with 10 mg metoclopramide orally 90 min preoperatively.

4. Monitoring

4.1 Standard monitoring

Heart rate and rhythm (electrocardiogram), noninvasive and direct arterial blood pressure measurement, pulse oximetry, end-tidal CO2, body temperature, urinary output, CVP, and neuromuscular blockade. Arterial blood gases, hematocrit, electrolytes, glucose, and serum osmolality should be measured periodically.

4.2 Monitoring for air embolism

Detection of venous air embolism by Doppler ultrasound should be considered for surgical procedures in which veins in the operative site are above the level of the heart.

4.3 Brain monitoring

Electroencephalogram, evoked potentials, jugular venous bulb oxygen saturation (Sjo2), flow velocity measured by transcranial Doppler (TCD), brain tissue Po2 (btPo2), and ICP may be used.

☐ The Sjo2 provides continuous information about the balance between global cerebral oxygen supply and demand. A Sjo2 of <50% for >15 minutes is a poor prognostic sign and is often associated with a poor neurologic outcome. The decrease in Sjo2 could be caused by excessive hyperventilation, decreased CPP, cerebral vasospasm, or a combination.

☐ Flow velocity of basal cerebral arteries as measured by the TCD technique is helpful in assessing the cerebral circulatory state at the bedside. However, it does not provide an absolute value for the CBF.

☐ Near-infrared spectroscopy, currently available in clinical practice, provides relative information about changes of oxy- and deoxy hemoglobin and the cytochrome oxidase redox status in the brain tissue of interest in a noninvasive and continuous fashion.

☐ ICP the association between severity of ICP elevation and poor outcome is well known.

Monitoring ICP is useful, therefore, not only as a guide to therapy, but also for assessing.

5. Intraoperative management

The major goals of anesthetic management are to (a) optimize cerebral perfusion and oxygenation, (b)) provide adequate surgical conditions for the neurosurgeons with a slack brain and low intracranial pressure (ICP). When a patient has an intracranial space occupying lesion (SOL), the achievement of a low ICP during surgery demands a careful choice of the most appropriate anesthetic and an attention to detail. A badly administered or inappropriate anesthetic may add to the intracranial problems generated by the space occupation, increasing ICP. General anesthesia is recommended to facilitate control of respiratory and circulatory function.

5.1 Factors that influence cerebral blood flow

PaO_2.

$PaCO_2$.

Cerebral metabolic rate.

☐ Arousal/pain.

☐ Seizures.

☐ Temperature.

☐ Anesthetics.

Blood pressure/status of auto regulation.

☐ Vasoactive agents

☐ Anesthetics.

☐ Pressers.

☐ Inotropes

5.2 The effects of anesthetics on intracranial and cerebral perfusion pressures

☐ Intravenous anesthetics:

Barbiturates. Thiopental and pentobarbital decrease CBF, cerebral blood volume (CBV), and

ICP. The reduction in ICP with these drugs is related to the reduction in CBF and CBV coupled with metabolic depression. These drugs will also have these effects in patients who have impaired CO_2 response.

Etomidate. As with barbiturates, etomidate reduces CBF, CMR_{O2}, and ICP. Systemic Hypotension occurs less frequently than with barbiturates. Prolonged use of etomidate may suppress the adrenocortical response to stress.

Propofol. The cerebral hemodynamic and metabolic effects of Propofol are similar to those of barbiturates. Propofol might be useful in patients who have intracranial pathology if hypotension is avoided. Because the context-sensitive half-life is short, emergence from anesthesia is rapid, even after prolonged administration. This may offer an advantage over other intravenous anesthetics in providing the opportunity for early postoperative neurologic evaluation. Because of propofol's potent circulatory depressant effect, recent studies have shown a reduction in jugular bulb oxygen saturation during Propofol anesthesia. Propofol can also reduce CBF more than CMR_{O2}, producing ischemia under certain conditions. Therefore, care should be taken when hyperventilating patients during Propofol anesthesia.

Benzodiazepines. Diazepam and midazolam may be useful either for sedating patients or inducting anesthesia because these drugs have minimal hemodynamic effects and are less likely to impair cerebral circulation. Diazepam, 0.1 to 0.2 mg/kg, may be administered for inducting anesthesia and repeated, if necessary, up to a total dose of 0.3 to 0.6 mg/kg.

Midazolam, 0.2 mg/kg, can be used for induction and repeated as necessary.

Narcotics.in clinical doses, narcotics produce a minimal to moderate decrease in CBF and

CMRo2. When ventilation is adequately maintained, narcotics probably have minimal effects on ICP. Despite its small ICP-elevating effect, fentanyl provides satisfactory analgesia and permits the use of lower concentrations of inhalational anesthetics. When these drugs are used, measures to maintain systemic blood pressure need to be implemented.

☐ Inhalational anesthetics:

Isoflurane has less effect on CBF and ICP than halothane has. Because isoflurane depresses cerebral metabolism, it may have a cerebral protective effect when the ischemic insult is not severe. Data favor the use of isoflurane over either halothane or enflurane. Isoflurane in concentrations of >1 minimum alveolar concentration should be avoided, however, because it can cause substantial increases in ICP.

Sevoflurane. Clinical studies have demonstrated, however, that sevoflurane's effect on cerebral hemodynamics is either similar to or milder than that of isoflurane. The disadvantage of Sevoflurane is that its biodegraded metabolite may be toxic in high concentrations. There is no evidence of an adverse effect at clinically used concentrations, however, unless Sevoflurane is administered in a low-flow circuit for prolonged periods.

Rapid emergence from anesthesia with Sevoflurane may be an advantage because it facilitates early postoperative neurologic evaluation.

Desflurane.

Desflurane at high concentrations appears to increase ICP.

Nitrous oxide (N2O). N2O dilates cerebral vessels, thereby increasing ICP. Patients who have intracranial hypertension or a decrease in intracranial compliance should, therefore, not receive this drug.

Local anesthetic. The infiltration of either lidocaine 1% or bupivacaine 0.25%, with or without epinephrine, in the skin around the scalp incision and the insertion sites for the pin head holder is helpful in preventing systemic and intracranial hypertension in response to these stimuli and avoiding the unnecessary use of deep anesthesia.

□ Muscle relaxants. Adequate muscle relaxation facilitates appropriate mechanical ventilation and reduces ICP. Coughing and straining are avoided because both can produce cerebral venous engorgement.

Vecuronium appears to have minimal or no effect on ICP, blood pressure, or heart rate and would be effective in patients with head injuries. This drug is given as an initial dose of 0.08 to 0.1 mg/kg followed by infusion at a rate of 1 to 1.7 mcg /kg /minute.

Pancuronium does not produce an increase in ICP but can cause hypertension and Tachycardia because of its vagolytic effect, thereby increasing the patient's risk.

Atracurium has no effect on ICP. Because of its rapid onset and short duration of action, a bolus dose of 0.5 to 0.6 mg/kg followed by a continuous infusion at a rate of 4 to 10 mcg/kg/minute is administered with monitoring of neuromuscular blockade.

Rocuronium is useful for intubation because of its rapid onset of action and lack of effect on intracranial dynamics. For maintenance, drugs with longer durations of action are recommended.

5.3 Induction

☐ Adequate preoperative anxiolysis in the anesthetic room

☐ Electrocardiogram, capnometer, pulse oximeter, noninvasive blood pressure

☐ Venous, arterial lines: insert under LA

☐ Furosemide 1 mg/kg

☐ Preoxygenation.

☐ Fentanyl, 1-2 mcg/kg, (alfentanil, sufentanil,and remifentanil),Propofol, 1.25-2.5 mg/kg, or thiopental, 3-6 mg/kg, then non depolarizing myo-relaxant

☐ Control ventilation (Paco2 ~ 35 mm Hg)

☐ Intubation. The airway should be secured with an armored endotracheal tube, taped on the contra lateral side to operation It may be desirable to secure the tube further using a throat pack. Careful taping is required to prevent both extubation and venous congestion.

5.4 Intraoperative respiratory management

5.5 Mechanical ventilation

Ventilation of the lungs is arranged so that there is a slow rate, with a long expiratory pause;

PEEP is normally not applied. A naso gastric tube should be considered for long operations.

Mechanical ventilation is adjusted to maintain a $Paco_2$ of around 35 mm Hg. The fraction of inspired oxygen (Fio_2) is adjusted to maintain a Pao_2 of >100 mm Hg.

5.6 Deliberate hypoventilation

Hypoventilation also increases cerebral blood flow and cerebral blood volume, which may impair surgical exposure. Until the benefits of hypoventilation are confirmed, mild hyperventilation is the more common practice.

Considerations of Brain Tumor Surgery

5.7 Position

Operations may last several hours so the patient should be carefully positioned with bony points padded, eyes protected with tape or gel and care taken to ensure tubing is not pressed against the patient's skin. Patients may be positioned supine or slightly rotated, with one shoulder raised, or they may be placed in a lateral position. A head-up tilt of the table of about 15° is essential to aid cerebral venous drainage. Pinealomas may be approached with the patient either prone or sitting.

A urinary catheter is necessary to assess fluid status. The patient's head position on the operating table is fixed either on a horseshoe type head rest or by the insertion of skull pins.

The application of the pins represents another stimulus causing an increase in blood pressure response, and great care should be taken to ensure that the patient is adequately anaesthetized before the pins are applied.

5.8 Maintenance of anesthesia

The ideal drug for maintenance of anesthesia should reduce ICP, maintain adequate oxygen supply to the brain tissue, and protect the brain against ischemic-metabolic insult. The selection of anesthetic drugs is based on a consideration of the intracranial pathology as wellas systemic conditions such as cardiopulmonary disturbances. There are different regimens can be used ,Isoflurane 1-2% versus Sevoflurane 0.5-1.5%– fentanyl 150 mcg/kg/min, or Desflurane 3-"6%, Propofol infusion- fentanyl, Propofol – remifentanil infusion, alfentanil, and sufentanil, and, and. neuromuscular blockade maintained using peripheral nerve stimulation.

5.9 Intraoperative hemodynamic management

CPP (cerebral perfusion pressure) should be maintained between 60 and 110 mm Hg. The transducer for direct monitoring of arterial blood pressure is zeroed at the level of mastoids to reflect the cerebral circulation.

5.10 Intravenous fluids

Intravenous fluids should be chosen with care; over transfusion will lead to a high CVP and therefore predispose to high ICP and use of solutions of glucose in water worsen cerebral edema. Patients with severe intracranial hypertension may have been drowsy or vomiting preoperatively and therefore may be hypovolemic. If mannitol has been used, fluids should be given to replace the deficit produced by diuresis. Mannitol may also produce hyponatraemia and hypokalemia. Normal saline or Hartmann's solution is indicated for fluid therapy during the procedure and should be given to replace fluid losses and controlled by the CVP to avoid over transfusion. Colloid solutions, such as modified gelatin (Gelofusine), may be given and blood loss over 1 liter should be replaced as appropriate.

5.11 Intra operative blood loss

Vascular tumors (notably meningiomas) can be associated with very fast blood loss and if the tumor is on the convexity of a cerebral hemisphere, the blood loss may occur during the cutting of the bone flap, when the surgeon may not be in a position to stop the bleeding. The anesthetist thus needs to have everything needed for rapid transfusion ready at the start of a craniotomy for a vascular tumor. Cross matched blood needs to be in the theatre suite and there must be a large-bore venous cannula in place, together with arterial and CVP measurement. A blood warmer needs to be set up and acid–base estimations available quickly. Further significant and persistent blood loss may occur during the subsequent resection of a meningioma, so it is important that the initial blood loss is replaced. The cerebral vasoconstriction that occurs with hemorrhage reduces CBF significantly, especially in the junctional areas between the major cerebral vessels.

5.12 Management intraoperative hypotension

Adequate oxygenation, ventilation, and fluid replacement, careful elevation of the blood pressure with a continuous infusion of an inotrope or vasopressor may be necessary.

Phenylephrine, 0.1 to 0.5 mcg/kg/minute, and dopamine, 1 to 10 mcg /kg/minute, are appropriate drugs in this setting. A bolus dose of vasopressor must be used cautiously because abrupt increases in blood pressure can elevate ICP to dangerous levels, especially in patients who have disordered auto regulation. Balance between maintenance of CPP to areas of brain rendered ischemic due to compression by hematoma, and the risk of more vasogenic brain edema or bleeding. Jugular venous bulb oxygen saturation monitoring may help assess adequacy of global.

5.13 Management intraoperative hypertension

Hypertension is treated cautiously because the elevation in blood pressure may reflect compensatory hyperactivity of the sympathetic nervous system in response to elevated ICP and compression of the brain stem (Cushing's reflex). Adequate oxygenation, ventilation, volume replacement, and analgesia should be first assessed and corrected. (i.e., opioids) and/or depth of anesthesia (Propofol, barbiturates, etomidate) before an antihypertensive drug, such as either labetalol or esmolol, which has minimal cerebral vasodilating effects, should be administered. When treating hypertension, maintenance of CPP is a major concern.

5.14 Induced hypotension

Hypotension to a MAP of 60–70 mmHg, which will provide a surgical field with reduced oozing, Before hypotension is used, the patient's physical state should be carefully assessed, particularly looking for signs of ischemia in the cerebral or coronary circulations or a history of hypertension. Hypotension should not normally be applied until the dura is open, and the length of hypotension should be kept as short as possible. Hypovolemia should not be allowed to coexist with induced hypotension; blood replacement must parallel blood loss.

CBF is maintained constant as long as the MAP is between 60 and 160 mmHg, may be of value.

Monitoring must be extensive and reliable; as well as the monitoring mentioned, jugular venous oxygen content measurements are valuable, as are transcranial Doppler measurements of flow velocity. The use of Propofol infusion with opioid analgesics and moderate hyperventilation provides a satisfactory surgical field for most neurosurgical operations but occasionally the resection of a large vascular tumor may still require hypotension. Hypotension is most easily induced by the combination of labetalol (10–20 mg) followed by sodium nitroprusside infusion (0.01%). The infusion is best given along the central venous line, so that the time lag between changing the infusion rate and observing the effect on blood pressure is kept to a minimum.

Sodium nitroprusside causes cerebral vasodilatation but the effect can be overcome by ensuring that the arterial pressure is lowered to at least 70% of the control value. If the anesthetic has been so arranged that the patient's cardiovascular system is stable and not responding to painful stimuli, hypotension should be easily achieved with such small doses of Propofol that toxicity is not invoked. If the patient develops a tachycardia or is resistant to sodium nitroprusside, it is better to supplement the action of sodium nitroprusside by another drug, such as labetalol or propranolol to control heart rate, or to increase the infusion of Propofol or the inhaled concentration of isoflurane, rather than using excessive

Infusion rates of sodium nitroprusside. Other hypotensive agents are available, such as trimetaphan and trinitroglycerine (GTN). GTN, like sodium nitroprusside, causes an increase in ICP and also a marked tachycardia. Trimetaphan is a less effective drug than either but does not because a rise in ICP, unless the patient is suffering from extreme degrees of intracranial space occupation, in which case the ganglionic blockade may produce an increase in CBF by blocking the sympathetic supply to the cerebral vessels.

When induced hypotension is being used, it is important that the surgeon knows this and that, after the tumor is resected, blood pressure is returned to normal before the dura is closed. This is essential so that the bleeding points can be visualized and sealed.

6. Tight brain (increased intracranial tension ICT)

6.1 Prevention

Preoperative: adequate anxiolysis and analgesia.

Pre induction: hyperventilate on demand, head-up position; head straight, no jugular vein compression.

Avoid over hydration.

Osmotic diuretics, as (mannitol, hypertonic saline); and steroids.

Loop diuretics (furosemide).

Optimize hemodynamics: MAP, central venous pressure, pulmonary capillary wedge pressure, and heart rate; use beta-blockers, clonidine, or lidocaine if necessary.

Ventilation: Pao2 >100; Paco2 ~ 35 mm Hg, low intra thoracic pressure.

Induction, and maintenance by use of intravenous anesthetics.

6.2 Treatment

Cerebrospinal fluid drainage (lumbar catheter or ventricle)

Osmotic diuretics.

Hyperventilation.

Augment depth of anesthesia using intravenous anesthetics (Propofol, thiopental,

Etomidate)

Muscle relaxation.

Improve cerebral venous drainage: head up, no positive end-expiratory pressure, reduce inspiratory time.

Mild controlled hypertension, if cerebral auto regulation intact (MAP ~ 100 mm).

7. Emergence from general anesthesia

The closure of a craniotomy may take a little time. Following surgery for a space-occupying lesion, some postoperative brains welling is likely and great care should be taken to ensure that the end of the anesthetic is smooth, without undue hypertension, coughing or straining.

☐ Movement of the head may take place then and the patient should not cough or strain. Normally, however, during the closure period, the Propofol and relaxant infusions can be reduced, the aim being to ensure that the patient is awake at the end of the procedure, but reversal of the muscle relaxant must be left until after any dressings or head bandages have been applied.

☐ avoiding of coughing and straining is essential. In order to avoid hypertension on extubation, removal of the endotracheal tube and suctioning of the pharynx may be covered with IV lignocaine 1.5 mg/kg 90 s before extubation. Labetalol can also be given to obtund these responses.

☐ Anesthetic technique should be so judged as to produce an awake, responding patient in the recovery area, so that neurological monitoring to detect the postoperative complications of hematoma formation may be started. 20% of elective craniotomy patients develop raised ICP in the early postoperative period. Systemic hypertension is frequent and has been associated with an increased risk of postoperative intracranial hemorrhage.

☐ Oxygen consumption is increased (up to 5 times) by re warming (shivering/ non shivering thermo genesis) and pain.

☐ Remifentanil can be used to control blood pressure during emergence of anesthesia after craniotomy for brain tumors. It has higher rapid recovery score than esmolol and other narcotics. In addition, it can be used when esmolol is contraindicated such as in cardiac patients, asthmatics, chronic obstructive pulmonary disease, or during pregnancy. Also, it decreases the need for postoperative analgesia and allows sedation if the infusion is continued as surgical patients are admitted to the ICU

7.1 Indications of postoperative intensive care unit after brain tumor surgery

1. Patients in whom a tight brain was present during surgery.

2. Excessive blood loss.

3. Edema spread is marked should be considered for postoperative pressure ventilation in an intensive care unit.

4. Obtunded consciousness

5. Inadequate airway control preoperatively;

6. Intraoperative catastrophe

7. Deranged intra cerebral hemo- or homeostasis postoperatively.

8. Long operation (>6 hours).

9. Repeated surgery,

10. Surgery involving or close to vital brain areas.

11. Surgery associated with significant brain ischemia (e.g., long vascular clipping times, extensive retractor pressure).

7.2 Differential diagnosis of unplanned delayed emergence

After 10 to 20 minutes of cessation of pharmacologically adequate anesthesia with short acting agents, the patient should be awake enough to obey simple verbal commands.

1. Opioid overhang (fentanyl or sufentanil): try carefully titrated antagonization with small doses of naloxone or naltrexone

2. Nonanesthetic causes (seizure, cerebral edema, intracranial hematoma, pneumocephalus, vessel occlusion/ischemia, metabolic or electrolyte disturbances).

8. Specific anesthetic considerations

8.1 Posterior fossa tumors

8.2 Positioning

☐ Prone postion:

This position offers good access to midline structures but bleeding can obscure the surgical field. Head-up tilt is employed to reduce hemorrhage but this increases the risk of air embolism. The head is fixed in clamps in preference to a horseshoe in order to minimize pressure on the face and eyes.

☐ Lateral position:

This is suitable for approaches to lesions not in the midline, particularly the cerebello pontine Angle. A pad should be placed under the body in the axilla to minimize weight on the lower arm and shoulder.

☐ sitting position:

This was widely used for posterior fossa surgery in the past.

Advantages of sitting position:

It provides good surgical access to midline structures,

Improves surgical orientation

It allows good Drains of blood, and CSF.

Complications of sitting position:

Cord compression.

Pneumocephalus. Following a craniotomy, an air-filled space between the dura, and arachnoids remains after CSF has leaked away during surgery, and brain bulk is reduced. In the recovery period brain bulk increases again as cerebral edema develops, arterial carbon dioxide concentrations increase and CSF re accumulates. The trapped air then comes under increasing pressure. N2O will worsen the situation. Pneumocephalus presents as delayed recovery or deteriorating neurological state and should always be considered if this occurs.

Pneumocephalus can be reduced by discontinuing nitrous oxide 15 minutes before surgery finishes and by allowing the PaCO2 to rise towards the end of surgery.

Venous air embolism.

The incidence of VAE during posterior fossa procedures in the sitting position is 40% to 45%. For seated cervical laminectomy or surgery in the prone or lateral positions, VAE occurs in approximately 10% to 15% of cases. VAE can occur whenever pressure within an open vessel is sub atmospheric. Clinically significant VAE is unusual unless the surgical site is >20 cm above the level of the heart.

When open vessels cannot collapse, which is the case with major venous sinuses as well as bridging and epidural veins, the risk of VAE increases substantially.

Massive air embolism produces abrupt and catastrophic hemodynamic changes.

Fortunately, this type of VAE is rare.

More commonly, air entrainment occurs slowly over a longer period of time and may produce little or no respiratory or hemodynamic compromise.

8.3 Monitoring for VAE

Hemodynamic changes. Monitoring of hemodynamics may not provide sufficient advanced warning in the case of massive air embolism because the hemodynamic changes are abrupt and catastrophic.

Doppler and ETco2 monitoring are considered the acceptable minimum.

Precordial Doppler

This device can detect 1 mL of air or less, which makes it more sensitive than any other monitor except Trans esophageal echocardiography (TEE). The Doppler is not quantitative, however, and it requires experience to recognize which of the various sounds it emits is indicative of air.

End-tidal gas monitoring VAE is associated with a decreasing ETco2 and the presence of end-tidal nitrogen (ETn2).

The CVP can help in positioning the Doppler. Also, the aspiration of air both confirms the diagnosis of VAE and serves as a treatment.

PA pressures rise with significant VAE, the PA catheter can be useful for both diagnosis and therapy.

Trans esophageal echocardiography (TEE) is more sensitive than Doppler ultrasound and is specific because the air bubbles are visualized directly.

8.4 Prevention of VAE

Positive end-expiratory pressure (PEEP)

☐ Use of PEEP to prevent VAE in the sitting position is controversial. High levels of
PEEP (>10 cm H2O) are needed to increase venous pressure at the head, and studies are inconsistent as to whether PEEP decreases the incidence of VAE. PEEP can, however, reduce venous return, cardiac output, and mean arterial blood pressure, which may be detrimental.

Volume loading

☐ Hypovolemia has been proposed as a predisposing factor for VAE.

☐ Deliberate hypoventilation

☐ Studies suggest that moderate hypoventilation may reduce the risk of
VAE, hypoventilation also increases cerebral blood flow and cerebral blood volume, which may impair surgical exposure.

9. Intraoperative anesthetic considerations of posterior fossa tumors

The conduct of anesthesia is similar to supratentorial surgery. Muscle relaxation is best provided by continuous infusion (e.g. Atracurium).This helps ventilation and prevents movement in a relatively lightly anesthetized patient. If motor nerve function is monitored, such as the facial nerve during acoustic neuroma surgery, Muscle relaxation must be discontinued, and sufficient depth of anesthesia must be provided. A remifentanil infusion is ideal in this situation. Hypotensive techniques increase the risks of ischemic damage specially in sitting position, and when the head is up position.

Hemodynamic instability occurs if the brainstem is manipulated. Bradycardia can occur when the peri ventricular grey matter and the reticular formation are stimulated. Most arrhythmias occur during surgery near the pons, and the roots of nerves V, IX and X.

Severe hypertension can result from stimulation of the trigeminal nerve.

9.1 Intraoperative brain stem monitoring

Monitoring techniques include somatosensory evoked potentials (SSEPs), brain stem auditory evoked potentials (BAEPs), and the spontaneous and evoked electromyogram

(EMG). This monitoring can be a challenge for the anesthesiologist because muscle relaxants complicate interpretation of the EMG, and N2O and high-dose inhalation anesthesia may interfere with SSEPs. Extubation should be delayed if there are concerns of brainstem or cranial nerve injury.

10. Post- operative special considerations after posterior fossa surgery

10.1 Ventilation/airway abnormalities

Because of disease- or surgery-induced dysfunction of cranial sensory or motor nerves, patients may have difficulty swallowing, vocalizing, or protecting the airway. In addition, damage to or edema of the respiratory centers from intraoperative manipulation can result in hypoventilation or erratic respiratory patterns. Therefore, longer-term ventilation and airway protection might be required in some patients.

Severe tongue and facial edema can occur owing to position-induced venous or lymphatic obstruction. The endotracheal tube should be left in place until the edema resolves.

Pulmonary edema may result from large VAE. Although pulmonary edema is usually responsive to conservative measures such as supplemental oxygen (O2) and diuretics, continued postoperative ventilation may be appropriate until evaluation is completed.

10.2 Cardiovascular complications

Hypertension is common after posterior fossa surgery and may contribute to edema formation and intracranial hemorrhage. Hence, one should be prepared to control postoperative hypertension.

10.3 Neurologic complications

A variety of untoward neurologic complications can occur after posterior fossa operations.

These include altered levels of consciousness, varying degrees of paresis, and specific cranial nerve deficits (e.g., visual disturbances, facial nerve paresis, impaired swallowing or phonation).

Treatment is supportive, but evaluation of delayed emergence should proceed lest a treatable non anesthetic cause go unrecognized. If cerebral paradoxical air embolism is suspected, hyperbaric oxygen therapy may be warranted.

Extreme neck flexion can cause mid cervical quadriplegia.

Peripheral nerve damage can result from faulty positioning. The brachial plexus, ulnar nerve and common peroneal nerve are most vulnerable.

10.4 Pneumocephalus

Air is retained in the cranial cavity after all craniotomies regardless of position. When the patient is in the sitting position, cerebrospinal fluid drains easily, and a larger amount of air may be trapped when the wound is closed. In most cases, the air is reabsorbed uneventfully over several days, and no treatment is necessary. There is little evidence that anesthetic technique influences either the incidence or the volume of pneumocephalus.

Tension pneumocephalus can occur when the brain re-expands and compresses the air. This situation is difficult to diagnose but should be suspected if emergence is delayed after an otherwise uneventful operation or if either cardiovascular collapse or neurologic deterioration occurs postoperatively. In such rare circumstances, surgical evacuation may be indicated

11. Trans sphenoidal hypophysectomy

The Trans sphenoidal approach to the pituitary is used for the excision of tumors that lie within the Sella or that has extension to the immediate supra sellar area.

11.1 Preoperative evaluation

Secreting lesions:

Prolactin Galactorrhea, a Cushing's disease (hypercortisolim, centripetal obesity, Diabetes mellitus, friable tissues .Acromegaly/gigantism, glucose intolerance, thick skin (difficult cannulation).

Non Secreting lesions:

Suprasellar Nonsecretory Panhypopituitarism, patients will commonly receive adrenal hormone supplementation at least temporarily. However, profound hypocortisolism with associated hyponatraemia should be corrected preoperatively.in fact uncommon for thyroid deficiency to occur. However, hypothyroidism should be sought and corrected preoperatively because hypothyroid patients have a diminished tolerance to the cardiovascular depressant effects of anesthetics. SIADH (syndrome of inappropriate antidiuretic hormone secretion), visual (optic chiasm) symptoms, Hydrocephalus may occur.

Monitoring:

Many practitioners place an arterial catheter, but it is not absolutely necessary. Access for blood sampling is a valuable adjunct to postoperative care if diabetes insipidus develops.

Blood loss is usually modest.

11.2 Anesthetic technique

The procedure is performed in a supine position, usually with some degree of head-up posture to avoid venous engorgement.

A pharyngeal pack will prevent an accumulation of blood in the stomach (which causes vomiting) or in the glottis (which contributes to coughing at extubation).

A RAE-type tube secured to the lower jaw at the corner of the mouth opposite the surgeon's dominant hand (e.g., the left corner of the mouth for a right-handed surgeon) is suitable.

A small esophageal stethoscope and temperature probe can lie with the endotracheal tube.

Covering the entire bundle with a towel drape (a plastic sheet with an adhesive edge) placed just below the lower lip so that it hangs from the lower jaw like a veil will protect it from the preparation solutions.

The procedure requires a C-arm image intensifier (lateral views), and the head and arms are relatively inaccessible once the patient is draped. It is appropriate to establish the nerve stimulator at a lower extremity site.

The surgical approach is through the nasal cavity by means of an incision made under the upper lip. During the approach, the mucosal surfaces within the nose are infiltrated with a local anesthetic and epinephrine solution, and the patient should be observed for the occurrence of dysrhythmias.

Surgical preferences for CO_2 management will vary. In some instances, hypocapania will be requested to reduce brain volume and thereby minimize the degree to which the arachnoid bulges into the sella.

Avoidance, when possible, of opening the arachnoid membrane. Postoperative CSF leaks can be persistent and are associated with a considerable risk of meningitis.

By contrast, in tumors with Suprasellar extension, normal or increased CO_2 will help deliver the lesion into the sella for excision. As an alternative method, some surgeons have resorted to "pumping" saline or air into the lumbar CSF space.

DI (Diabetes insipidus) usually develops 4 to 12 hours postoperatively and very rarely arises intraoperatively. The clinical picture is one of polyuria in association with a rising serum osmolality. The diagnosis is made by comparison of the osmolality of urine and serum.

Hyperosmolar urine in the face of an elevated and rising serum osmolality strongly supports the diagnosis. Desmopressin (DDAVP) is usually administered. In general, the patient is losing fluid that is hypoosmolar and relatively low in sodium. Half-normal saline and 5% dextrose in water (D5 W) are commonly used as replacement fluids.

12. Awake craniotomy

Awake craniotomies are performed when tumors or epileptic foci lie close to the cortical areas required for either speech or motor function or close to the mesial temporal structures critical to short-term memory.

12.1 Pre anesthetic Evaluation/Preparation

At the preoperative interview, the patient should be educated about the nature and duration of the procedure and the limitations on movement. One should obtain a description of both the aura and the seizures to facilitate recognition of them. One should a certain whether the patient is subject to grandmal convulsions.

If intraoperative electrocorticography to identify seizure foci is intended, it is common to discontinue or reduce the anticonvulsant dose by half according to the perceived risk of uncontrolled seizures.

Premedication drugs with an anticonvulsant effect, such as the benzodiazepines, should not be used because they may interfere with intraoperative EEG localization

12.2 The objectives of the anesthetic technique are to

Minimize patient discomfort associated with the potentially painful portions of the procedure, and with the prolonged restriction of movement.

Ensure patient responsiveness and compliance during the phases of the procedure that require assessment of either speech or motor/sensory responses to cortical stimulation.

Select anesthetic techniques that produce minimal inhibition of spontaneous seizure activity.

There are probably many ways of providing sedation that are consistent with the mentioned objectives, and many techniques are in active use. They range from minimal sedation approaches, through deep sedation during which intermittent unresponsiveness is achieved with spontaneous ventilation and an unprotected airway, to asleep-awake-asleep techniques with intermittent airway management with an LMA(laryngeal mask air way), sometimes with positive-pressure ventilation.

12.3 Anesthetic techniques

An awake craniotomy is the surgeon's local anesthetic technique. "Sedation" cannot compensate for inadequate anesthesia of the scalp, as accomplished with pin site infiltration and nerve blocks.

Typically, this procedure is performed as (a monitored anesthesia care) "MAC," although small doses of induction anesthetic, most often Propofol, are usually required at the time of stimulation of the periosteum at the base of the skull by the needle.

After placement of the relevant electrodes, the patient's seizure medication is discontinued and the patient remains in an observation unit with EEG and patient behavior recorded continuously. In this manner, the EEG events associated with the clinically significant seizure events and their anatomic origin can be identified.

Several centers have used a droperidol/synthetic narcotic combination (e.g., droperidol, 2.5 to 7.5 mg; alfentanil, 5- to 10-mg/kg load, 0.5- to 1.0-mg/kg/min infusion; Fentanyl, 0.7- mg/kg load, 0.7- mg/kg/hr infusion).

Others use principally propofol by either physician- or patient-controlled infusion.

Care should be taken when administering additional sedative agents, especially narcotics, whose respiratory depressant effects might be synergistic with propofol. This consideration is especially relevant when pin fixation is used. Pin fixation severely restricts the Anesthesiologist's capacity to intervene quickly in the event of excessive respiratory depression or loss of patency of the airway.

Propofol, if used, should be discontinued at least 15 minutes before EEG recording. In spite of prompt awakening, propofol leaves a residual EEG "footprint" characterized by high frequency, high-amplitude beta activity that can obscure the abnormal activity that is being sought in the cortical surface EEG. Various groups have reported use of the LMA, commonly with narcotic-propofol sedation and spontaneous ventilation during the craniotomy; administration of the sedative is discontinued and the LMA is removed once the brain surface is exposed.

Infusion of remifentanil and propofol and positive-pressure ventilation.

More recently, the α2 -agonist dexmedetomidine at low dose (0.1 to 0.3 mg/kg/hr) has been used by some, both with and without intermittent use of the LMA.

12.4 Monitoring during awake craniotomy

Routine, noninvasive monitors are almost always sufficient. Reliable capnography to provide breath by-breath confirmation of airway patency and respiratory drive is an essential component of the technique if deep sedation is intended for any portion of the procedure. These procedures are often lengthy, and attention to the details of patient comfort (warming blankets, a sheepskin, and room temperature) will improve patient tolerance.

13. References

[1] Nicolas J. Bruder, Patrick A. Ravussin.Anesthesia for Supratentorial Tumors, Handbook of Neuroanesthesia, 4th Edition, 2007 Lippincott Williams & Wilkins.

[2] Patterson JT, Hobnail F, Franklin RL, Nauta HJW. Neurosurgey. In: Townsend CM, Beauchamp RD, Evers BM, Mattox KL, eds. *Sabiston Textbook of Surgery.* 18th ed. Philadelphia, Pa: Saunders Elsevier; 2007:chap 72.

[3] Michael F. Roizen; Preoperative Evaluation ,: Miller's Anesthesia, 6th ed., Copyright © 2005 ELSEVIER CHURCHILL LIVINGSTONE.

[4] John C. Drummond,Piyush M. Patel Neurosurgical Anesthesia Miller's Anesthesia, 6th ed., Copyright © 2005 ELSEVIER CHURCHILL LIVINGSTONE.

[5] Richard A, Girard F, Girard DC, et al. Cisatracurium-induced neuromuscular blockade is affected by chronic phenytoin or carbamazepine treatment in neurosurgical patients. Anesth Analg 2005;100:538â€"544.

[6] Petersen KD, Landsfeldt L, Cold GE, et al: Intracranial pressure and cerebral hemodynamics in patients with cerebral tumors: A randomized prospective study of patients subjected to craniotomy in propofol-fentanyl,isoflurane-fentanyl, or sevoflurane-fentanyl anesthesia. Anesthesiology 98:329, 2003.

[7] Hernandez-Palazon J, Martinez-Lage JF, Rosa-Carrillo VN, et al: Anesthetic technique
and development of pneumocephalus after posterior fossa surgery inthe sitting position. Neurocirurgia 14:216, 2003.

[8] Kaisti KK, Langsjo JW, Aalto S, et al. Effects of sevoflurane, propofol, and adjunct nitrous oxide on regional cerebral blood flow, oxygen consumption, and blood volume in humans. Anesthesiology 2003;99:603-613.

[9] Goma HM, Ali MZ Control of emergence hypertension after craniotomy for brain tumor surgery. Neurosciences (Riyadh). 2009 Apr;14(2):167-71.

[10] Yoshimitsu K, Suzuki T, Muragaki Y, Chernov MIseki H. Development of modified
Intraoperative Examination Monitor for Awake Surgery (IEMAS) system for awake craniotomy during brain tumor resection. Conf Proc IEEE Eng Med Biol Soc.
2010;1:6050-3.

[11] Tsuruta S, Yamada M, Shimizu T, Satsumae T, Tanaka M, Mizutani T. Airway management using i-gel in two patients for awake craniotomy. Masui. 2010
Nov;59(11):1411-4.

[12] Andersen JH, Olsen KS .Anaesthesia for awake craniotomy is safe and well-tolerated. Dan Med Bull. 2010 Oct;57(10):A4194.

[13] Wu CT, Chen LC, Kuo CP, Ju DT, Borel CO, Cherng CH, Wong CS.A comparisonof 3% hypertonic saline and mannitol for brain relaxation during elective supratentorial brain tumor surgery. Anesth Analg. 2010 Mar 1;110(3): 903-7.

[14] Sharma D, Ellenbogen RG, Vavilala MSUse of transcranial Doppler ultrasonography and jugular oximetry to optimize hemodynamics during pediatric posterior fossa craniotomy. J Clin Neurosci. 2010 Dec;17(12):1583-4. Epub 2010 Aug 25.

[15] Kassebaum N, Hairr J, Goldsmith W, Barwise J, Pandharipande PDiabetes insipidus associated with propofol anesthesia. . Clin Anesth. 2008 Sep;20(6):466-8.